I0791204

**ISBN:** 9781677573165

# 7-DAY
# GLUTEN FREE
# EXPRESS DIET

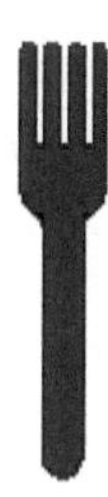



## Gail Johnson, M.S.

NoPaperPress™

# CONTENTS

Gluten is a mixture of two proteins that are present in wheat, barley and rye. Gluten causes harmful reactions to people who have celiac disease or are gluten sensitive. But gluten is difficult to avoid, because wheat is the third largest crop in the U.S. (behind corn and soybeans). When the acreage for wheat, barley and rye are combined, more farm acres are used to grow gluten grain crops than any other, with about 4 billion bushels of gluten grains grown in 2011. Because wheat, barley and rye grains are everywhere in our food chain, eating gluten-free involves more complicated than just substituting gluten-free bread for the usual gluten-containing bread for sale on supermarket shelves.

Another problem is gluten cross contamination which occurs when a gluten-free food comes in contact with a food that contains gluten. Cross contamination can happen at a farm where the food is grown, at a manufacturing facility where the food is processed, at a supermarket where a food may be re-packaged, and in your kitchen.

Gluten-free means that a food does not contain the gluten in wheat, barley or rye and sometimes cross-contaminated oats or soy.

## Why Gluten Free?

The primary reason for a gluten-free diet is to combat celiac disease which is a chronic, systemic, autoimmune disorder that causes intestinal damage. For more on celiac disease see **Appendix A**, page 37.

Another reason to go gluten free is to combat a condition called non-celiac gluten sensitivity that can also affect nearly every system in your body with symptoms that include digestive complaints, skin problems, brain fog, joint pain and numbness in extremities. Still another reason for a gluten-free diet is to combat a wheat allergy. For more on non-celiac gluten sensitivity see Appendix A.

A new reason to go gluten free is that many adults claim that going gluten free not only helped them lose weight but they also felt a lot better. For more on this again see Appendix A.

## Is This Diet For You?

The *7-Day Gluten-Free Express Diet* is for adult men and women:
- **Who just want to lose weight and feel better on a gluten-free diet.**
- **With gluten sensitivity or a wheat allergy who want to lose weight.**
- **With celiac disease who want to lose weight.**

The low-calorie menus assure that you will lose weight, while going gluten free is a healthy bonus that also makes many people feel better while on the diet.

## Choose Your Calorie Level

This eBook contains two 7-day diets: a 1,200-Calorie diet and a 1,500-Calorie diet.  And both diets have a meal plan (menu) for each and every one of the 30 days.  Which diet calorie level should you choose?

**<u>1,200-Calorie Diet</u>** is **appropriate for most women**.  But due to the relatively low calorie level, you might occasionally feel hungry.  (The 1,500-Calorie diet might be a better choice for some larger, younger, or more active women.)

**<u>1,500-Calorie Diet</u>** is **suitable for most men**.  This is a reasonable diet calorie level where most adults easily get all the nutrients and micro nutrients they need – and rarely feel hungry.  (The 1,200-Calorie diet might be a better choice for some smaller, or older, or inactive men.)

## Expected Weight Loss

Weight loss  occurs when your food energy intake is less than the total energy you expend. This difference in calories is referred to as your <u>calorie deficit</u>. How much weight you lose depends on the magnitude of your calorie deficit.  Physiologists have long known that to lose one pound requires a deficit of approximately 3,500 Calories. Therefore, if a person's total calorie deficit over time is known, their weight loss over time can be calculated.

On the *7-Day Gluten-Free Express Diet*, **<u>most women lose 3 to 4 pounds.</u>**  Smaller women, older women and less active women lose a bit less and larger women, younger women and more active women often lose more.

On the *7-Day Gluten-Free Express Diet*, **<u>most men lose 4 to 5 pounds.</u>**  Smaller men, older men and less active men will lose a tad less and larger men, younger men and more active men much more.

If you want to lose even more weight take a brisk one-hour walk every day.  This applies to both men and women.

Exactly how much weight you will lose depends on how much you weigh, your age and your activity level.  For the full story see *Weight Control - U.S. Edition* by Vincent W. Antonetti, Ph.D.

## How to Use This eBook

**1)**  Read material in **Appendix A** (page 37):  "Gluten Notes" and **Appendix B**: (page 40) which lists "Gluten-Free Foods."

**2)**  Choose the calorie level that's right for you, either 1200 or 1500 Calories per day - depending on your gender, your size, age and how active you are.

**3)**  Then to start the diet go to either:

**Day 1 of the 1200-Calorie Diet** (page 14)

**Day 1 of the 1500-Calorie Diet** (page 22)

## First a Medical Exam

Even though this diet adheres to the United States Department of Agriculture balanced diet recommendations, it may not be appropriate for everyone, such as individuals with illnesses such as heart disease, diabetes, etc. Make sure you check with your physician before starting this diet, or any diet. **Everyone should at the very least have a medical assessment, or exam, before starting a weight loss diet.** Why? You need to make sure your health will allow you to lower your caloric intake and increase your physical activity. Depending on your age and state of health, the medical checkup may be as simple as a visit to a physician who is familiar with your medical history, or it may be a thorough physical exam.

The physician conducting the medical exam should be made aware of and should approve the specific weight loss diet you're planning. Additionally, if you are going to engage in some sort of physical activity in conjunction with this diet and especially if you have been totally inactive, or if you have or suspect you have cardiovascular disease or other health problems, or if you are obese, or if you are 40 or older, before embarking on the physical fitness portion of your weight control program you should have a stress test supervised by a physician. Finally, your physician can tell you how much and what type of exercise is right for you, how much you should weigh, and prescribe a realistic weight- loss goal.

## Eat Smart – Gluten Free

First, please read **Appendix B** (page 40) "Gluten-Free Foods" which is a listing of many of the gluten-free foods that are available in supermarkets and online.

Then understand that no single food can supply all the nutrients you need in the amounts you need. Gluten free aside for the moment, the most important factors in nutrition are variety, variety, variety! **Variety is the key to a nutritious diet.** As a means of setting strategies for food selection, the U.S. Department of Health and Human Services and the Department of Agriculture issue Dietary Guidelines every five years. The latest Dietary Guidelines describe a healthy diet as one that:
- Emphasizes fruits, vegetables, whole grains, and fat-free or low-fat milk products.
- Includes fish, poultry, lean meats, beans and nuts.
- Is low in saturated fats, trans fats, cholesterol, salt (sodium) and added sugars.

The latest guidelines encourage adults to consume a variety of nutrient-dense foods and beverages within their caloric needs. The afore mentioned U.S. government agencies recommend how much should be eaten from each of the basic food groups.  For detailed information on gluten-free eating see **Appendix B** (page 40).

Even though most adults can get all the vitamins and minerals they need by merely consuming a variety of nutritious foods (from the fruit group, the vegetable group, the grains group, the meat and beans group, the milk group, and the oils group), many physicians recommend a daily multi-vitamin/mineral supplement – just in case you don't eat the way you should.

Be aware that some micronutrients, such as the fat-soluble vitamin A, can be harmful if taken in large quantities.  To be safe your multi-vitamin/mineral supplement should contain no more than 100 percent of the recommended dietary allowance (RDA) for each vitamin or mineral. Generally, you don't need the high doses in multi-vitamin/mineral supplements labeled "therapeutic" or "extra-strength."  There may be medical reasons for taking larger amounts of a vitamin or mineral than the RDA provides, but check with your doctor first.

## Tossed Salad

One of the dinner mainstays of the *7-Day Gluten-Free Express Diet* is a gluten-free "Tossed Salad."  To prepare your "Tossed Salad" start with a bowl that has a volume of <u>at least</u> 16 ounces, or 2 cups.  First add about 1 cup of either green-leaf lettuce, Romaine lettuce or a Mesclun mix.  Then add at least a half cup of other veggies such as broccoli, celery, cucumber, spinach, or watercress.  This vegetable combination will, on average, total about 35 Calories.

You'll be eating a "Tossed Salad" just about every day at dinnertime. Remember that variety is the key to a nutritious diet.  So be sure to vary the ingredients of the salad.  Top your "Tossed Salad" with <u>1½ tablespoons of a gluten-free lite salad dressing</u> that contains no more than 25 Calories per tablespoon.  Some of our favorite gluten-free light salad dressings are:
- **Annie's Lite Raspberry Vinaigrette**
- **Ken's Lite Options Italian w/ Romano & Red Pepper**
- **Newman's Own Lite Red Wine Vinaigrette & Olive Oil**
- **San-J's Tamari Sesame Salad Dressing**

For more gluten-free salad dressing options see page 47.  Your "Tossed Salad" with gluten-free salad dressing will cost you roughly 70 Calories but will be packed with lots of health-giving vitamins, minerals and fiber.

## About Bread

First appreciate that bread, more specifically whole-grain breads, are good sources of complex carbohydrates and dietary fiber, as well as the B vitamins (thiamin, riboflavin, niacin, and folate), vitamin E, and minerals (iron, magnesium and selenium).  The gluten in wheat, barley and rye consists of two proteins that combine during baking to develop a substance that provides bread with elasticity and structure.  Gluten also helps bread dough rise into a light loaf.  Other grains do not have these characteristics, which is why it is difficult to find good gluten-free bread.

The *7-Day Gluten-Free Express Diet* requires bread at about 70 Calories per slice.  These days many supermarkets stock gluten-free bread. The difficult part is finding a good tasting gluten-free bread with about 70 Calories per slice.  The gluten-free bread at your local supermarket vary in taste and texture, so try different brands before deciding.  As of this writing, our favorite gluten-free bread is Udi's, particularly Udi's Whole-Grain Bread at about 65 Calories per slice.

## Substituting Foods

If there is a food listed in the diet that you don't like, or perhaps that you forgot to pick up while shopping, you probably can exchange or substitute another food in its place – a technique used by dieticians.  Exchanging a food listed in a diet for another food with approximately equal caloric value and nutritional content is the foundation of many successful long-term diets. Substitution possibilities are almost endless but have to be done carefully. The easiest substitutions are those within the same food group, such as exchanging one vegetable variety for another, or a glass of milk for a cup of yogurt.  More sophisticated exchanges cross food groups, such as replacing 3½ ounces of turkey with a tablespoon of peanut butter on a piece of whole-wheat bread. Both foods are complete protein and both contain about 175 Calories.  With some understanding and experience, you can substitute foods called for in this diet with equal calorie foods from the same food group.

**Breakfas**t: You may substitute any cereal for any other gluten-free cereal.  For example, if you're not crazy about having Kellogg's Rice Krispies - gluten-free for breakfast on Day 4, substitute General Mills Corn Chex, etc.  But remember to adjust the amount of cereal to account for the calorie difference between brands.  (See page 40 for a list of gluten-free cereals.)  And if you don't like the scrambled egg called for on Day 1, have a soft-boiled egg instead.  And if Cantaloupe is on the menu but is not in season, replace cantaloupe with a half cup of orange juice – both contain about 50 Calories.

**Snacks**: Again, where 6 ounces of yogurt is specified you may substitute an 8-ounce glass of skim milk, but to maintain a nutritionally balanced diet keep this snack a dairy selection.  Similarly, when fruit is on the menu, you may select any type of fruit but do not stray from the fruit group.  Nuts and popcorn can be interchanged at will.  Specified convenient brand-name snacks, such as Skinny Cow ice cream bars and Orville

Redenbacher's Smart Pop Popcorn should be widely available but other equivalent brands may be substituted if need be.  Just make sure the substitute snack has the same calorie count, or very close, to the specified snack.

## Important Notes

**1)**  If desired, skim milk and a sugar substitute may be added to coffee or tea. And soy or almond milk may be used instead of cow's milk.

**2)**  Fried eggs and scrambled eggs should be cooked in a pan coated with a non-stick cooking spray.  DO NOT USE butter or oil.

**3)**  On bread, corn-on-the-cob, or a baked potato, if desired, you may use a zero-calorie butter substitute spray.  (I Can't Believe It's Not Butter spray is gluten free.) DO NOT USE butter or sour cream.

**4)**  Cereals should be selected from the following gluten-free varieties: General Mills Rice Chex, General Mills Corn Chex, General Mills Vanilla Chex, General Mills Cinnamon Chex, General Mills Chocolate Chex, General Mills Apple Cinnamon Chex, General Mills Honey Nut Chex, Glutino Honey Nut, Glutino Apple Cinnamon, Kellogg's Rice Krispies - gluten-free, Bob's Red Mill Oat Meal and Gifts of Nature (Montana) Oat Meal.

**5)**  Bread:  Udi's Whole Grain Bread is a good choice and has 65 Calories per slice. These days many supermarkets stock gluten-free bread although you often can find a better selection online.  If desired, bread may be sprayed with a zero-calorie butter substitute.  DO NOT USE butter.

**6)**  Use only lean cuts of meat trimmed of all visible fat.  Poultry should be limited to chicken or turkey breasts (white meat and skinless only).

**7)**  When canned tuna or salmon is specified, use only fish packed in water.

**8)**  An unlimited amount of green salad may be eaten, but the GF salad dressing should be as specified on page 9.  (Note, in the meal plans Evoo means extra virgin olive oil.)

**9)**  Use freely as desired: clear unsweetened coffee, clear unsweetened tea, water, seltzer water, any diet soda, clear soups without fat, bouillon, and seasonings such as mustard, cinnamon, dill, herbs, red and black pepper, curry and vinegar.

**10)**  Any specified snack may be moved to any other part of the day, and/or combined with lunch or dinner.

**11)**  After you complete the 7th day on the diet, if you still want to lose more weight you may repeat the diet by starting over at Day 1.

## Keeping It Off

Within five years, more than 90 percent of all dieters regain every pound they have lost.  Why?  In most cases it's because after losing weight most people eventually revert to their pre-diet eating and exercising habits, and this

inevitably leads to their regaining the weight they lost – and often more. Obviously after a diet you weigh less.  The fact is the less you weigh, the less you need to eat to sustain your lower weight.

A study, published in the *Annals of Internal Medicine*, that followed 4,000 people for three decades suggests that in the long term, 90 percent of men and 70 percent of women will become overweight.  Interestingly, half of the men and women in the study, who had made it well into adulthood without a weight problem, ultimately also became overweight and a third actually became obese.  The point being that you can never become complacent.  You must continually watch your weight because we are all at risk of becoming overweight.

The key to long-term weight control success is knowledge and understanding, combined of course with desire and self-discipline.  Once you reach your weight goal, we suggest you read ***Weight Maintenance - U.S. Edition*** by Vincent Antonetti, Ph.D. (also published by NoPaperPress) – absolutely the best weight maintenance book, or eBook, on the market.

# 1200 Calorie Meal Plans

# Day 1 - 1200 Calorie Meal Plan

| BREAKFAST | Calories | Totals |
|---|---|---|
| Grapefruit (½) | 75 | |
| Scrambled egg | 80 | |
| Gluten-free bread (page 40) toasted (1 slice) | 70 | |
| Coffee (Notes - page 11) | 10 | 235 Cal |
| | | |
| **SNACK** | | |
| Coffee or tea | 10 | 10 Cal |
| | | |
| **LUNCH** | | |
| Ham* (2 oz) with mustard on 2 slices GF bread | 290 | |
| Pickle spear | 0 | |
| Small bunch of grapes | 65 | |
| Hot or iced tea | 10 | 365 Cal |
| | | |
| * See page 45. | | |
| **SNACK** | | |
| Fresh fruit in season (apple, peach, etc) | 70 | |
| Coffee or tea | 10 | 80 Cal |
| | | |
| **DINNER** | | |
| Chicken w Peppers & Onions (Day 1 Recipe  page 30) | 250 | |
| Sautéed red peppers with onions (Day 1 recipe) | 70 | |
| Green beans - steamed | 25 | |
| Mashed cauliflower | 30 | |
| Large tossed salad w 1½ Tbsp lite GF dressing (p 47) | 70 | |
| Skim milk (4 ounces - ½ cup) | 45 | 490 Cal |
| | | |
| **SNACK** | | |
| Coffee or tea | 10 | 10 Cal |
| | | |
| | | 1195 Cal |

# Day 2  1200 Calorie Meal Plan

| BREAKFAST | Calories | Totals |
|---|---|---|
| Orange juice (½ cup) | 50 | |
| Rice Chex* (1 cup) + ½ cup skim milk + ½ sliced banana | 195 | |
| Coffee (Notes - page 11) | 10 | 255 Cal |
| | | |
| * See page 41 for more GF cereals. | | |
| **SNACK** | | |
| | | |
| Fresh fruit in season (apple, pear, etc) | 70 | |
| Coffee or tea | 10 | 80 Cal |
| | | |
| **LUNCH** | | |
| | | |
| Soup # 10 (Appendix C - page 49) | 110 | |
| GF turkey breast* (1 oz) on 1 slice GF bread | 120 | |
| Pickle spears | 0 | |
| Lettuce & tomato slices | 20 | |
| Water | 0 | 250 Cal |
| | | |
| * See page 45. | | |
| **SNACK** | | |
| | | |
| Coffee or tea | 10 | 10 Cal |
| | | |
| **DINNER** | | |
| | | |
| Baked Herb-Crusted Cod (Day 2 Recipe - page 31) | 230 | |
| Spinach (½ cup) steamed w garlic & drizzled w Evoo | 100 | |
| Asparagus (8 spears cooked & drained) | 25 | |
| Baked potato (medium - No Butter!) | 100 | |
| Gluten-free (GF) bread* (1 slice) | 70 | |
| Water with lemon wedge | 10 | 535 Cal |
| * See page 40. | | |
| **SNACK** | | |
| | | |
| GF Cookie (page 43) | 60 | |
| Coffee or tea | 10 | 70 Cal |
| | | |
| | | 1200 Cal |

# Day 3  1200 Calorie Meal Plan

| BREAKFAST | Calories | Totals |
|---|---|---|
| Fresh or frozen strawberries (½ cup) | 25 | |
| French toast (Day 3 Recipe - page 32) | 310 | |
| GF Lite Syrup* (1 Tbsp) | 30 | |
| Coffee | 10 | 375 Cal |
| * See page 48. | | |
| **SNACK** | | |
| Coffee or tea | 10 | 10 Cal |
| | | |
| **LUNCH** | | |
| Salad (3 oz canned tuna* 1 tsp Evoo onions celery) | 175 | |
| Lettuce & tomato wedges | 20 | |
| GF bread (1 slice) | 70 | |
| Fresh fruit in season (apple, peach, etc) | 70 | |
| Coffee or tea | 10 | 345 Cal |
| * See page 45. | | |
| **SNACK** | | |
| Coffee or tea | 10 | 10 Cal |
| | | |
| **DINNER** | | |
| Broiled veal chop (4 oz lean) | 200 | |
| Corn on the cob (1 medium ear) (No Butter!) | 100 | |
| Broccoli (½ cup steamed & drizzled with 1 tsp | 70 | |
| Large tossed salad w 1½ Tbsp lite GF dressing (p | 70 | |
| Water with lemon wedge | 10 | 450 Cal |
| | | |
| **SNACK** | | |
| Coffee or tea | 10 | 10 Cal |
| | | |
| | | 1200 Cal |

# Day 4  1200 Calorie Meal Plan

| BREAKFAST | Calories | Totals |
|---|---|---|
| Grapefruit (½) | 75 | |
| Rice Krispies* (1 cup) + ½ cup milk+ 1 Tbsp raisins | 200 | |
| Coffee | 10 | 285 Cal |
| | | |
| * Gluten-free variety | | |
| **SNACK** | | |
| Coffee or tea | 10 | 10 Cal |
| | | |
| **LUNCH** | | |
| GF Cottage cheese* (1 cup no fat) | 140 | |
| Tossed salad with 1½ Tbsp lite GF dressing (page | 70 | |
| GF bread (1 slice) | 70 | |
| Hot or iced tea | 10 | 290 Cal |
| | | |
| * Cabot No-Fat Cottage Cheese is gluten free.  See page 46. | | |
| **SNACK** | | |
| Fresh fruit in season (peach, plum, etc) | 70 | |
| Coffee or tea | 10 | 80 Cal |
| | | |
| **DINNER** | | |
| Meat Loaf (Day 4 Recipe - page 33) | 290 | |
| One-half acorn squash (baked w ½ tsp maple | 90 | |
| Spinach (½ cup steamed & drizzled with 1 tsp Evoo) | 70 | |
| Lettuce, tomato slices & 1 Tbsp lite GF dressing | 45 | |
| Water | 0 | 495 Cal |
| | | |
| * Pure maple syrup is naturally gluten free | | |
| **SNACK** | | |
| GF Ginger-Snap Cookie (page 43) | 40 | |
| Coffee or tea | 10 | 50 Cal |
| | | |
| | | 1210 Cal |

# Day 5  1200 Calorie Meal Plan

| BREAKFAST | Calories | Totals |
|---|---|---|
| Orange juice (½ cup) | 50 | |
| Cinnamon Chex* (¾ cup) + ½ cup milk + ½ banana | 215 | |
| Coffee | 10 | 275 Cal |
| | | |
| * See page 41 for more GF cereals. | | |
| **SNACK** | | |
| | | |
| Fresh fruit in season (apple, plum, etc) | 70 | |
| Coffee or tea | 10 | 80 Cal |
| | | |
| | | |
| **LUNCH** | | |
| Leftover meat loaf  (½ of Day 4 serving size) w | 155 | |
| GF bread (1 slice) | 70 | |
| Lettuce | 10 | |
| Fresh or frozen berries (½ cup) | 50 | |
| Hot or iced tea | 10 | 295 Cal |
| | | |
| **SNACK** | | |
| | | |
| Handful of unsalted mixed nuts (page 46) | 100 | |
| Coffee or tea | 10 | 110 Cal |
| | | |
| **DINNER** | | |
| | | |
| Margherita Pizza (Day 5 Recipe - page 34) | 230 | |
| Large tossed salad with 1½ Tbsp lite GF dressing | 70 | |
| Water with lemon wedge | 10 | 310 Cal |
| | | |
| **SNACK** | | |
| | | |
| Skinny Cow Chocolate Truffle Bar (ice cream*) | 100 | |
| Coffee or tea | 10 | 110 Cal |
| | | |
| * See page 46. | | 1180 Cal |

# Day 6  1200 Calorie Meal Plan

| BREAKFAST | Calories | Totals |
|---|---|---|
| Cantaloupe (½ medium) | 50 | |
| Rice Chex (1 cup) + ½ cup skim milk + ½ banana | 195 | |
| Coffee | 10 | 255 Cal |
| | | |
| **SNACK** | | |
| Fresh fruit in season (peach, plum, etc) | 70 | |
| Coffee or tea | 10 | 80 Cal |
| | | |
| **LUNCH** | | |
| Soup (Appendix C - page 49) | 140 | |
| GF turkey breast* (1 oz) on 1 slice GF bread | 120 | |
| Lettuce & tomato slices | 20 | |
| Hot or iced tea | 10 | 290 Cal |
| | | |
| **SNACK** | | |
| Coffee or tea | 10 | 10 Cal |
| | | |
| **DINNER** | | |
| Baked salmon with salsa (Day 6 Recipe - page 35) | 215 | |
| Baked summer squash and zucchini | 40 | |
| Medium tomato - sliced | 20 | |
| Brown rice* (½ cup – after cooking) | 100 | |
| Large tossed salad with 1½ Tbsp lite GF dressing | 70 | |
| Water with lemon wedge | 10 | 455 Cal |
| | | |
| * See page 44. | | |
| **SNACK** | | |
| GF Popcorn - 100 Calorie Mini Bag (page 46) | 100 | |
| Coffee or tea | 10 | 110 Cal |
| | | |
| | | 1200 Cal |

# Day 7  1200 Calorie Meal Plan

| BREAKFAST | Calories | Totals |
|---|---|---|
| Orange juice (½ cup) | 50 | |
| Cinnamon Chex (1 cup) + ½ cup milk + ½ banana | 255 | |
| Coffee | 10 | 315 Cal |
| | | |
| **SNACK** | | |
| Handful of unsalted mixed nuts (page 46) | 100 | |
| Coffee or tea | 10 | 110 Cal |
| | | |
| **LUNCH** | | |
| GF Turkey Hot Dog* with mustard & relish | 100 | |
| GF Hot-dog bun** | 150 | |
| Diet soda or water | 0 | 250 Cal |
| | | |
| * See page 45.   ** See page 40. | | |
| **SNACK** | | |
| Coffee or tea | 10 | 10 Cal |
| | | |
| **DINNER** | | |
| Pasta with Marinara sauce (Day 7 Recipe - page 36) | 225 | |
| Large tossed salad with 1½ Tbsp lite GF dressing | 70 | |
| Fresh fruit in season (peach, plum, etc) | 70 | |
| GF bread (1 slice) | 70 | |
| Water with lemon wedge | 10 | 445 Cal |
| | | |
| **SNACK** | | |
| GF Cookie (page 43) | 60 | |
| Coffee or tea | 10 | 70 Cal |
| | | |
| | | 1200 Cal |

# 1500 Calorie Meal Plans

# Day 1 - 1500 Calorie Meal Plan

| BREAKFAST | Calories | Totals |
|---|---|---|
| Grapefruit (½) | 75 | |
| Scrambled egg | 80 | |
| GF Turkey bacon* (1 slice) | 35 | |
| Gluten-free bread (GF bread)** toasted (1 slice) | 70 | |
| Coffee (Notes - page 11) | 10 | 270 Cal |
| * See page 45.   ** See Page 40. | | |
| **SNACK** | | |
| GF yogurt - page 46  (6 oz, nonfat, any flavor) | 90 | |
| Coffee or tea | 10 | 100 Cal |
| **LUNCH** | | |
| Ham* (2 oz) with mustard on 2 slices GF bread | 290 | |
| Pickle spear | 0 | |
| Small bunch of grapes | 65 | |
| Hot or iced tea | 10 | 365 Cal |
| * See page 45. | | |
| **SNACK** | | |
| Fresh fruit in season (apple, peach, etc) | 70 | |
| Coffee or tea | 10 | 80 Cal |
| **DINNER** | | |
| Chicken w Peppers & Onions (Day 1 Recipe  page 30) | 250 | |
| Sautéed red peppers with onions (Day 1 recipe) | 70 | |
| Green beans - steamed | 25 | |
| Mashed cauliflower | 30 | |
| Large tossed salad with 1½ Tbsp lite GF dressing* | 70 | |
| GF bread** (1 slice) | 70 | |
| Skim milk (4 oz - ½ cup) | 45 | |
| Water with lemon wedge | 10 | 570 Cal |
| | | |
| * See page 47. ** See page 40. | | |
| **SNACK** | | |
| GF Popcorn - 100 Calorie Mini Bag (page 46) | 100 | |
| Coffee or tea | 10 | 110 Cal |
| | | 1495 Cal |

# Day 2  1500 Calorie Meal Plan

| BREAKFAST | Calories | Totals |
|---|---|---|
| Orange juice (½ cup) | 50 | |
| Rice Chex* (1 cup) + ½ cup milk+ ½ banana | 195 | |
| GF bread toasted (1 slice) | 70 | |
| Coffee | 10 | 325 Cal |
| | | |
| * See page 41 for more GF cereals. | | |
| **SNACK** | | |
| Fresh fruit in season (apple, pear, etc) | 70 | |
| Coffee or tea | 10 | 80 Cal |
| **LUNCH** | | |
| Soup (Appendix C - page 49) | 110 | |
| GF turkey breast* (1 oz) on 1 slice GF bread | 120 | |
| Pickle spear | 0 | |
| Lettuce & tomato slices | 20 | |
| Water | 0 | 250 Cal |
| | | |
| * See page 45. | | |
| **SNACK** | | |
| GF Popcorn - 100 Calorie Mini Bag (page 46) | 100 | |
| Coffee or tea | 10 | 110 Cal |
| **DINNER** | | |
| Baked Herb-Crusted Cod (Day 2 Recipe - page 31) | 230 | |
| Spinach (½ cup) steamed with garlic & drizzled | 100 | |
| Asparagus (8 spears cooked & drained) | 25 | |
| Baked potato (medium - No Butter!) | 100 | |
| Gluten-free (GF) bread (1 slice) | 70 | |
| Water with lemon wedge | 10 | 535 Cal |
| | | |
| **SNACK** | | |
| Raw Revolution Peanut Butter Chocolate Bar* | 200 | |
| Coffee or tea | 10 | 210 Cal |
| * See page 43. | | |
| | | 1510 Cal |

# Day 3  1500 Calorie Meal Plan

| BREAKFAST | Calories | Totals |
|---|---|---|
| Fresh or frozen strawberries (½ cup) | 25 | |
| French toast (Day 3 Recipe - page 32) | 310 | |
| GF Lite Syrup* (1 Tbsp) | 30 | |
| Coffee | 10 | 375 Cal |
| | | |
| * See page 48. | | |
| **SNACK** | | |
| GF yogurt - page 46  (6 oz, nonfat, any flavor) | 90 | |
| Coffee or tea | 10 | 100 Cal |
| | | |
| **LUNCH** | | |
| Salad (3 oz canned tuna*, 1 tsp Evoo, onions, celery) | 175 | |
| Lettuce & tomato wedges | 20 | |
| GF bread (1 slice) | 70 | |
| Fresh fruit in season (apple, peach, etc) | 70 | |
| Coffee or tea | 10 | 345 Cal |
| | | |
| * See page 45. | | |
| **SNACK** | | |
| Handful of unsalted mixed nuts (page 46) | 100 | |
| Coffee or tea | 10 | 110 Cal |
| | | |
| **DINNER** | | |
| Broiled veal chop (4 oz lean) | 200 | |
| Corn on the cob (1 medium ear) (No Butter!) | 100 | |
| Broccoli (½ cup steamed & drizzled with 1 tsp | 70 | |
| Large tossed salad w 1½ Tbsp lite GF dressing (p 47) | 70 | |
| Water with lemon wedge | 10 | 450 Cal |
| | | |
| **SNACK** | | |
| Skinny Cow Chocolate Truffle Bar (ice cream*) | 100 | |
| Coffee or tea | 10 | 110 Cal |
| * See page 46. | | |
| | | 1490 Cal |

# Day 4  1500 Calorie Meal Plan

| BREAKFAST | Calories | Totals |
|---|---|---|
| Grapefruit (½) | 75 | |
| Rice Krispies* (1 cup) + ½ cup milk+ 1 Tbsp raisins | 200 | |
| GF bread toasted (1 slice) | 70 | |
| Coffee | 10 | 355 Cal |
| | | |
| * Gluten-free variety | | |
| **SNACK** | | |
| | | |
| Fresh fruit in season (peach, plum, etc) | 70 | |
| Coffee or tea | 10 | 80 Cal |
| | | |
| **LUNCH** | | |
| GF Cottage cheese* (1 cup no fat) | 140 | |
| Large tossed salad w 1½ Tbsp lite GF dressing (p 124) | 70 | |
| GF bread (1 slice) | 70 | |
| Hot or iced tea | 10 | 290 Cal |
| | | |
| * Cabot No-Fat Cottage Cheese is gluten free | | |
| **SNACK** | | |
| | | |
| Handful of unsalted mixed nuts (page 46) | 100 | |
| Coffee or tea | 10 | 110 Cal |
| | | |
| **DINNER** | | |
| | | |
| Meat Loaf (Day 4 Recipe - page 33) | 290 | |
| One-half acorn squash (baked with ½ tsp maple | 90 | |
| Spinach (½ cup steamed & drizzled with 1 tsp Evoo) | 70 | |
| Romaine lettuce, tomato slices & 1 Tbsp lite GF | 45 | |
| Water | 0 | 495 Cal |
| | | |
| * Pure maple syrup is naturally gluten free. | | |
| **SNACK** | | |
| | | |
| Two GF Oatmeal-Raisin Cookies (page 43) | 180 | |
| Coffee or tea | 10 | 190 Cal |
| | | |
| | | 1520 Cal |

# Day 5  1500 Calorie Meal Plan

| BREAKFAST | Calories | Totals |
|---|---|---|
| Grapefruit (½) | 75 | |
| Cinnamon Chex (¾ cup) + ½ cup milk + ½ banana | 215 | |
| Toasted GF bread (2 slices) | 140 | |
| Coffee | 10 | 440 Cal |
| | | |
| **SNACK** | | |
| Handful of unsalted mixed nuts | 100 | |
| Coffee or tea | 10 | 110 Cal |
| | | |
| **LUNCH** | | |
| Leftover meat loaf  (½ of Day 4 serving) w ketchup | 155 | |
| GF bread (1 slice) | 70 | |
| Lettuce | 10 | |
| Fresh fruit in season (apple, peach, etc) | 70 | |
| Hot or iced tea | 10 | 315 Cal |
| | | |
| **SNACK** | | |
| GF Popcorn - 100 Calorie Mini Bag | 100 | |
| Coffee or tea | 10 | 110 Cal |
| | | |
| **DINNER** | | |
| Margherita Pizza (Day 5 Recipe page 34) | 230 | |
| Large tossed salad w 1½ Tbsp lite GF dressing (p 47) | 70 | |
| Water with lemon wedge | 10 | 310 Cal |
| | | |
| **SNACK** | | |
| Raw Revolution Peanut Butter Chocolate Bar* | 200 | |
| Coffee or tea | 10 | 210 Cal |
| | | |
| * See page 43. | | 1495 Cal |

# Day 6  1500 Calorie Meal Plan

| BREAKFAST | Calories | Totals |
|---|---|---|
| Cantaloupe (½ medium) | 50 | |
| Rice Chex (1 cup) + ½ cup milk* + ½ banana | 215 | |
| Coffee | 10 | 275 Cal |
| | | |
| * Use skim milk. | | |
| **SNACK** | | |
| | | |
| Fresh fruit in season (peach, plum, etc) | 70 | |
| Coffee or tea | 10 | 80 Cal |
| | | |
| **LUNCH** | | |
| | | |
| Soup (Appendix C - page 49) | 140 | |
| GF turkey breast* (1 oz) on 1 slice GF bread | 120 | |
| Lettuce & tomato slices | 20 | |
| Hot or iced tea | 10 | 290 Cal |
| * See page 45. | | |
| **SNACK** | | |
| | | |
| GF Popcorn - 100 Calorie Mini Bag | 100 | |
| Coffee or tea | 10 | 110 Cal |
| **DINNER** | | |
| | | |
| Baked salmon with salsa (Day 6 Recipe page 35) | 215 | |
| Baked summer squash and zucchini | 40 | |
| Medium tomato - sliced | 20 | |
| Brown rice* (½ cup – after cooking) | 100 | |
| Large tossed salad with 1½ Tbsp lite GF dressing | 70 | |
| GF bread (1 slice) | 70 | |
| Water with lemon wedge | 10 | 525 Cal |
| | | |
| * See page 44. | | |
| **SNACK** | | |
| | | |
| Raw Revolution Peanut Butter Chocolate Bar | 200 | |
| Coffee or tea | 10 | 210 Cal |
| | | |
| | | 1490 Cal |

# Day 7  1500 Calorie Meal Plan

| BREAKFAST | Calories | Totals |
|---|---|---|
| Orange juice (½ cup) | 50 | |
| Cinnamon Chex (1 cup) + ½ cup milk + ½ banana | 255 | |
| GF bread - toasted (1 slice) | 70 | |
| Coffee | 10 | 385 Cal |
| | | |
| **SNACK** | | |
| Handful of unsalted mixed nuts | 100 | |
| Coffee or tea | 10 | 110 Cal |
| | | |
| **LUNCH** | | |
| GF Turkey Hot Dog* with mustard & relish | 100 | |
| GF Hot-dog bun** | 150 | |
| Diet soda or water | 0 | 250 Cal |
| | | |
| * See page 45.  ** See page 40. | | |
| **SNACK** | | |
| GF Popcorn - 100 Calorie Mini Bag | 100 | |
| Coffee or tea | 10 | 110 Cal |
| | | |
| **DINNER** | | |
| Pasta w Marinara sauce (Day 7 Recipe - page 36) | 225 | |
| Large tossed salad with 1½ Tbsp lite GF dressing | 70 | |
| Fresh fruit in season (peach, plum, etc) | 70 | |
| GF bread (1 slice) | 70 | |
| Water with lemon wedge | 10 | 445 Cal |
| | | |
| **SNACK** | | |
| Two GF Cookies* | 180 | |
| Coffee or tea | 10 | 190 Cal |
| | | |
| * See page 43. | | 1490 Cal |

# Recipes and Diet Tips

# Day 1- Recipe

## <u>Day 1 - Chicken with Peppers & Onions</u>

   4 boneless and skinless chicken breasts (about 5 oz each)

Coat the chicken breasts in a bottled barbeque sauce.  Prepare medium-hot fire on well-oiled grill.  Place breasts on grill, turning them every 4 minutes, for 10 to 12 minutes, or until done.  (To check if breasts are done, the meat should be moist and white with no sign of pink when you cut into the breast.)  Salt and pepper to taste.

   2  medium red peppers, sliced

   1  medium onion, sliced

Place peppers and onions in pan with 2 tablespoons fat-free **gluten-free chicken stock** (page 48).  Sauté until stock is reduced.  Spray pan lightly with **non-stick cooking oil** (page 46) and cook another 2 minutes.  Salt and pepper to taste.

<u>Serves 4</u>.  About 250 Calories per serving (for chicken only).

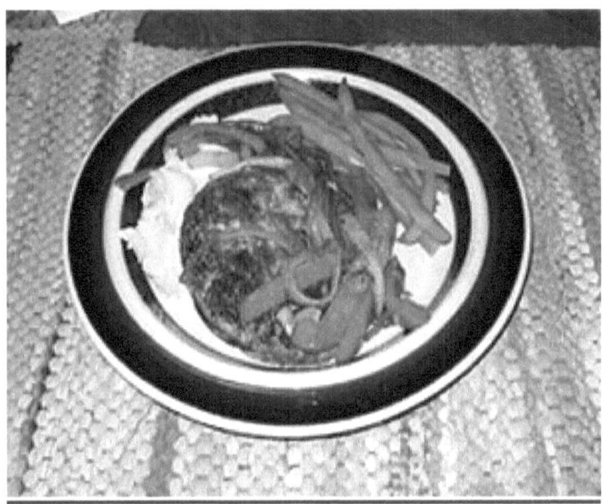

<u>Diet Tip of the Day:</u>  Weight Loss – take it one step, one meal, one workout, one day at a time.  Just think of where you'll be in 90 days!

# Day 2 - Recipe

## <u>Day 2 - Baked Herb-Crusted Cod</u>

- 4  cod fish fillets (4 to 5 ounces each)
- 2  tablespoons **all-purpose GF free flour** (page 40)
- 2  tablespoons GF cornmeal
- 2  tablespoons minced fresh herbs
- 2  teaspoons lemon juice

Sprinkle cod with lemon juice.  Mix flour, cornmeal and herbs and dust the cod with the cornmeal-herb mixture.  Bake in oven at 375 ºF for 10 minutes. Add salt and black pepper to taste.

<u>Serves 4</u>.  One serving is about 230 Calories (for cod only).

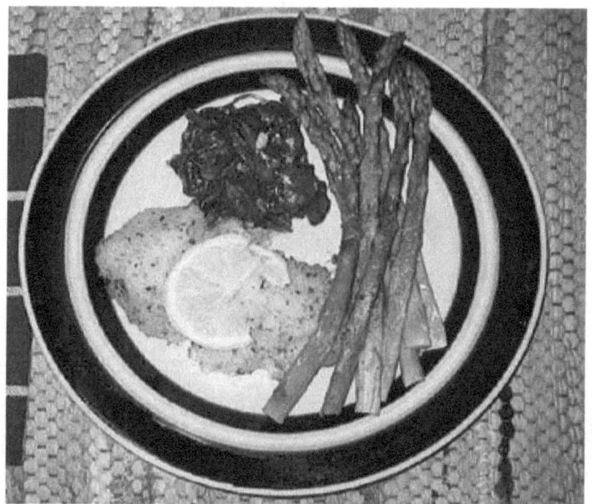

<u>Diet Tip of the Day:</u>. A **reducing diet is best supervised by a physician**. This is especially true when a great deal of weight needs to be lost, or if you have an ailment or a history of medical problems.

# Day 3 - Recipe

## Day 3 - French-Toast

   6 slices **GF bread** (page 40)
   2 eggs
   ⅓ cup skim milk
   1 teaspoon vanilla
   A dash of cinnamon

In a medium bowl, beat together eggs and skim milk.  Add vanilla and cinnamon.  Saturate bread slices in egg mixture.  In a non-stick skillet coated with a **GF cooking oil spray** (page 46), cook bread slices until both sides are golden brown.  If desired, dust lightly with confectionary sugar.  Serve hot or keep in an oven or warmer at 200 °F until ready to plate.

**Serves 2**.  Three slices of French toast per serving.  Each serving is 310 Calories.

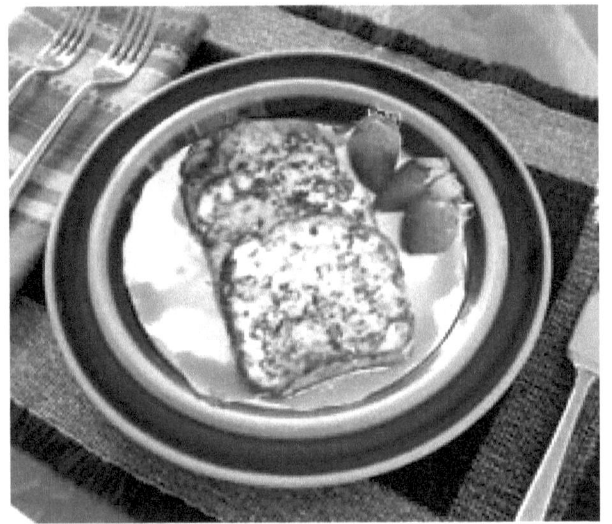

**Diet Tip of the Day:** **"Eat Slowly"**  This is especially vital when you are trying to lose weight.  If you are someone who eats fast, who finishes before everyone else at the table, you are not giving yourself a chance to feel full.  While everyone else is still eating, you either sit there and pick, or you have seconds, taking in extra calories you could avoid if you would just slow down.

* We prepared this dish using Udi's gluten-free whole grain bread.  Delicious!

## Day 4 - Recipe

## <u>Day 4 - Carrie's Low-Cal Meat Loaf</u>

½ pound ground white meat turkey
½ pound ground beef (about 90% lean)
1 large egg
½ cup skim milk
¼ cup GF bread crumbs (page 40)
¼ cup ketchup
¼ cup chopped carrots
¼ cup chopped onion

In a medium bowl, combine all ingredients.  Add salt and pepper to taste.
Mix until blended and form into a loaf.  Place loaf into oven preheated to 350
°F.  Bake until an instant-read thermometer inserted in the center of the loaf
reads 160 °F.  This should take about one hour.

Shown below is meat loaf, acorn squash (baked with 1 teaspoon of pure
maple syrup).  Also shown is steamed spinach drizzled with extra-virgin
olive oil.

<u>Serves 5</u>.  About 290 Calories per serving (for meat loaf only).  Note: reserve
half a serving of the meat loaf which is to be eaten for lunch on Day 6.

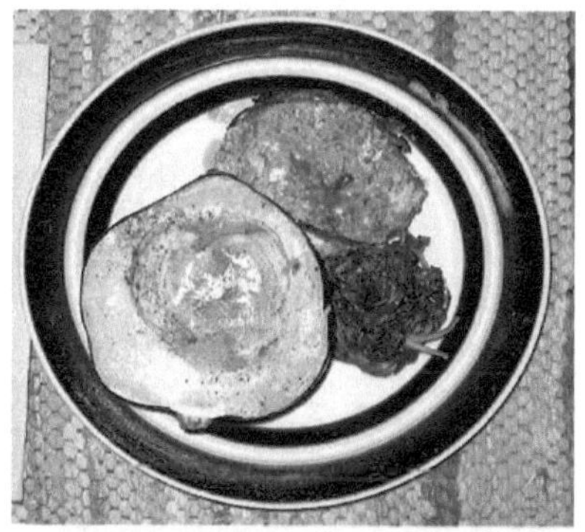

<u>Diet Tip of the Day:</u>  Get a **pedometer** and start walking.  For the average
person 2,100 steps amounts to walking about one mile.  A Harvard study has
shown that 8,000 to 10,000 step per day promote weight loss.  And you're not
obliged to walk continuously until you accrue all 10,000 steps.  Rather, all
steps throughout the day to wherever and whenever count toward your daily
total.  Because 10,000 steps a day may not be achievable by some people,
particularly those who are elderly, sedentary, or who have chronic diseases,
rather than insisting on a blanket 10,000 steps per day, your initial stepping
goal should your baseline steps plus an increment of an additional 2,500
steps. (Your baseline being the number of steps you take in an average day.)

## Day 5 - Margherita Pizza

In the original 7-Day Diet we featured a pizza recipe used by Gail Johnson's Italian grandmother.  From feedback, our readers thought it was absolutely delicious - they loved it.  We tried hard to make the pizza gluten free but just couldn't get the same crust and taste.  After testing several commercially available brands of gluten-free pizza crust and finally settled on the following recipe (which makes two 9-inch pizzas):

- 1   medium onion, minced & 1 clove of garlic, minced
- ¼   teaspoon dry oregano & ⅓.cup fresh basil leaves, torn
- 3   oz part-skim mozzarella cheese, shredded
- 2½ cups whole peeled canned tomatoes (page 42)
- 1   tablespoon extra-virgin olive oil, divided
- 2   9-inch diameter GF pizza crust*

**Tomato Sauce**: Over medium high heat, sauté minced onion in two teaspoons of olive oil.  Then stir in garlic, oregano, salt and pepper and ¼ teaspoon crushed red pepper (optional)..  Add tomatoes including most of the juice in the can, crushing them as you put them in pan.  Add ½ cup of water and simmer until sauce is reduced by one-half.

Brush one side of pizza crust with about a teaspoon of olive oil.  Spread tomato sauce over  crust and sprinkle shredded mozzarella cheese on top.  Place pizza on the lower rack of an oven preheated to 375ºF.  Cook approximately 15 minutes or until cheese melts and bottom of pizza crust is brown.  Sprinkle with fresh basil leaves.  Cut and serve.

**Serves 4**.  230 Calories per serving.  One full pizza shown below but a serving is half of a pizza.

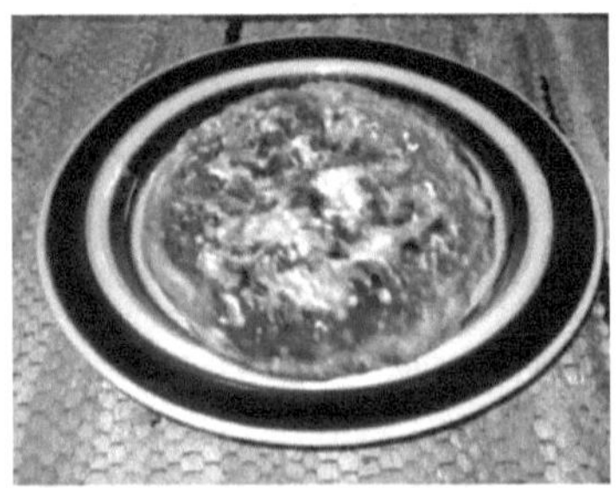

* We used Udi's GF Pizza Crust - 8 oz pkg which contains two 9-inch pizza crusts.

**Diet Tip of the Day:**  For **life-long weight control** take a vigorous 30 to 60 minute walk everyday!  That's right – everyday.  Make exercise a nonflexible top priority part of your life.  When it comes to exercise the key words are consistent, persistent, unyielding, dogged.  Get the point?

## Day 6 - Baked Salmon with Salsa

This is a simple, straight-forward recipe.  The advantage of a simple recipe is there are no hidden calories.

4   5 oz salmon fillets

6   tablespoons bottled salsa*

Brown salmon fillets in non-stick pan and then place them in a baking dish. Cook fillets in an oven preheated to 350 ºF for about 10 minutes.  Plate the salmon.  Stir bottled tomato-pepper salsa and spoon it over the salmon. **Serves 4**.  One salmon fillet is about 215 Calories.

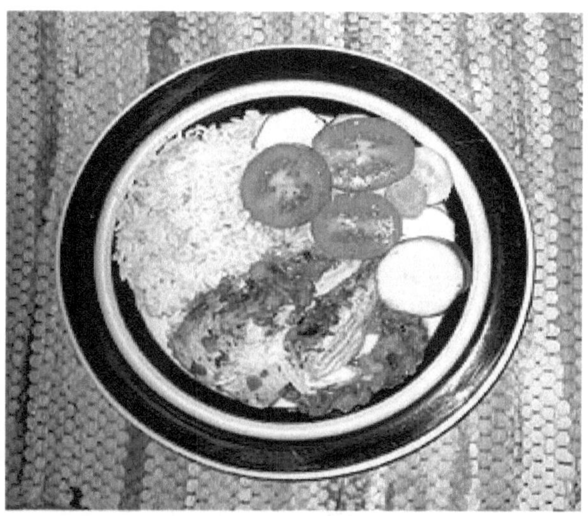

* We used Ortega's Garden Vegetable GF salsa.  See page 42 for other gluten-free salsas.

**Diet Tip of the Day:** Hunger is your body's way of telling you that you need calories. But **when you're done eating, you should feel better – satisfied but not stuffed**.

# Day 7 - Recipe

## <u>Day 7 - Pasta with Marinara Sauce</u>

The spiral pasta profile shown below is called fusilli, a very popular pasta shape because all those ridges hold lots of tomato sauce.

    ½ small onion, finely chopped
    1 teaspoon olive oil
    2 garlic cloves, finely chopped
    1½ cups chopped plum tomatoes
    ½ teaspoon chopped fresh oregano
    ½ pound gluten-free fusilli pasta*
    ¼ teaspoon salt

**Homemade Tomato sauce:**  Sauté chopped onion in 1 teaspoon olive oil. Add two finely chopped garlic cloves, 1½ cups chopped plum tomatoes and ½ teaspoon chopped fresh oregano.  Stir and cook about 5 minutes on a low flame.

**Pasta**: Bring 2 quarts of lightly salted water to a boil.  Add GF pasta and stir occasionally (to keep pasta from sticking to the bottom of the pot).  Keep water boiling and cook until pasta are "al dente."  (Cooking time is about 9 minutes.)  Because the tomato sauce is a bit too thick, add ¼ cup of pasta liquid to the sauce to thin it.  Finally drain the pasta, add the marinara sauce and serve hot.

<u>Serves 4.</u>  One serving is about 250 Calories.

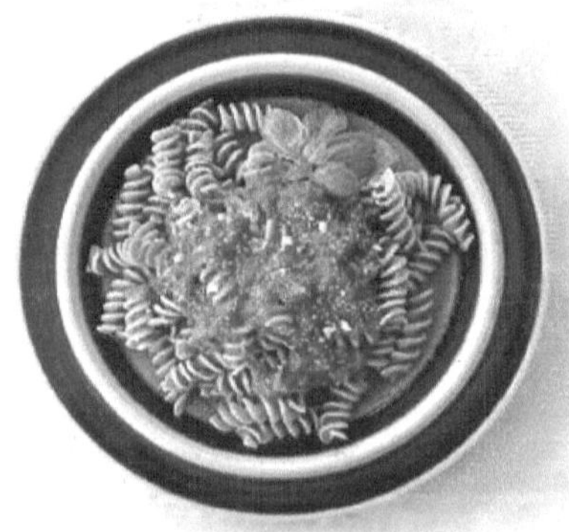

* We used Delallo Whole Grain Rice Fusilli.  Chef, Gail Johnson said, "DeLallo pasta is very good with a nice bite and an agreeable flavor."  See page 46 for additional gluten-free pasta choices.

<u>Diet Tip of the Day:</u>  **Beware of alcoholic beverages**.  Beer has about 13 Calories per ounce, wine 25 Calories per ounce and whiskey a whopping 71 Calories per ounce.

# Appendix A
# Gluten Notes

**Celiac Disease**:  The primary reason for a gluten-free diet is to combat celiac disease which is a chronic, systemic, autoimmune disorder that causes intestinal damage.  Common celiac symptoms include diarrhea, abdominal pain, weight loss and fatigue.  On the other hand, some celiac suffers experience constipation instead of diarrhea, weight gain instead of weight loss and heartburn instead of stomach pain.  And a few people diagnosed with celiac disease have almost no symptoms.  In net, celiac affects many body systems in different ways and because every person displays celiac disease differently, it is a difficult condition to diagnose.  A strict gluten-free diet most often alleviates celiac-related symptoms.  Keep in mind that all of these possible celiac disease symptoms can be caused by other medical problems.  If you suspect you have celiac disease, make sure to see a physician.

**Non Celiac Gluten Sensitivity**:  Another reason to go gluten free is to combat a condition called non-celiac gluten sensitivity that can also affect nearly every system in the body with symptoms that include digestive complaints, skin problems, brain fog, joint pain and numbness in extremities. Because research into this condition is in its early stages, not all physicians have accepted it as an illness and as a result not all physicians provide patients with a diagnosis of gluten sensitivity.  Nevertheless, if you believe you suffer from gluten sensitivity, see a physician.  To make matters even more confusing, some people are allergic to wheat.  These people experience typical allergy symptoms (nasal congestion, etc) and sometimes they also have gastrointestinal symptoms.

**Healthier Way to Lose Weight**:  A new reason to go gluten free is that some medical practitioners believe it is a healthier way to lose weight.  But gluten-free weight loss is a recent concept and to date there has not been any research that confirms going gluten free promotes weight loss.  Many physicians, however, report a considerable number of their patients claim that when they went gluten free they lost weight and felt a lot better.

**Gluten Restriction Levels**:  Because people with celiac disease and gluten sensitivity have remarkably varying degrees of reaction to trace levels of gluten, it is useful to think in terms of three levels of gluten restriction:

 The <u>first level</u> consists of adults with celiac disease.  These individuals have a medical reason for being on a gluten-free diet and have serious reactions to gluten.  They should avoid not only obvious gluten-laden foods, but also should avoid processed foods that have trace amounts of gluten as well as gluten-free foods that have been cross-contaminated by gluten foods or by trace gluten.  (The obvious gluten-laden foods include bread, cereals, and all products with wheat, barley or rye as an ingredient.)

The <u>second level</u> of gluten restriction consists of individuals with non-celiac gluten sensitivity or a wheat allergy who may or may not have a reaction to trace gluten in their food.  These people should avoid the obvious gluten containing foods and by trial and error learn what supposedly gluten-free foods (that nevertheless might contain trace gluten) they should also avoid.

In the <u>third level</u> are those who only want to lose weight and feel better on a gluten free diet.  These people have only to avoid obvious gluten-containing foods.

**Eating Gluten Free in Brief**:  First, you should be aware of food label ingredients that mean that gluten grains are present:  these are triticum vulgare (wheat), triticum spelta (a form of wheat), triticale (cross between wheat and rye), hordeum vulgare (barley) and secale cereale (rye).

Any of the following ingredients on a label indicate that the food definitely contains gluten: wheat protein, hydrolyzed wheat protein, wheat starch, hydrolyzed wheat starch, wheat flour, bread flour, bleached flour, bulgur (a form of wheat), malt (made from barley), couscous (made from wheat), farina (made from wheat), pasta (made from wheat unless otherwise indicated), seitan (made from wheat gluten and commonly found in vegetarian meals) and wheat germ oil or extract (likely cross contaminated).

Any of the following on a label indicate that the food might contain gluten: vegetable protein, hydrolyzed vegetable protein (could be from wheat, corn or soy), modified starch, modified food starch (can come from several sources, including wheat), natural flavor (can be made from barley), artificial flavor (can come from barley), modified food starch, hydrolyzed plant protein (HPP), hydrolyzed vegetable protein (HVP), seasonings, flavorings, vegetable starch, dextrin (sometimes made from wheat) and maltodextrin (sometimes made from wheat).

If a product contains wheat, the FDA requires that it be stated on the food's label. But other gluten-containing grains (barley or rye) do not have to be declared although they might have been added to a food's ingredients. If in doubt, check with the food manufacturer to determine if a food is truly gluten free. (Incidentally, when you call a manufacturer, it is not unusual for them to offer discount coupons for their products!)

**Gluten Cross Contamination**:  Of course, a food that has no gluten-containing ingredients could be cross contaminated with gluten.  For example, soybeans and oats do not naturally contain gluten.  But soybeans and oats are frequently grown in rotation with wheat crops. That means farmers often use the same fields to grow soy, oats  and wheat, they use the same combines to harvest the crops, the same storage facilities and the same trucks to transport the crops to market.  As a result, soy and oats are often gluten cross-contaminated.

So if you react to a food that is not supposed to have any gluten ingredients, it is probably because the food contains trace gluten due to cross contamination. The food might have just enough trace gluten to give you problems, despite having an apparently safe list of ingredients.

Appreciate that reactions to gluten vary from person to person. And a gluten reaction is influenced not only by how much gluten is in a food, but also by how much of that food you eat.

**Gluten-Free Labeling Standards**: The quantity of gluten in a particular product is expressed as parts of gluten contained in a million parts of the product, stated as parts per million, or ppm of gluten.  In 2013, the U.S. Food and Drug Administration allowed food manufacturers to label products "gluten-free" that contain less than 20 ppm of gluten (GF 20). Canada the UK and most European Union countries also consider 20 ppm to be gluten free. (20 ppm means a product contains 0.002% gluten).  Some people, however, still react to products labeled "gluten-free" that contain less than 20 ppm of gluten.  Because of this, several food manufacturers maintain more rigorous standards, typically lowering the amount of gluten in a product to less than 5 or 10 ppm.

# Appendix B
# Gluten-Free Foods

Because food ingredients and formulations can change at any time, the following lists and recommendations should only be used as a guide. Read the food label and ingredient statement on the food package carefully at the time of purchase to ensure it is gluten free. Moreover, recall that only people with celiac disease and those with extreme gluten sensitivity usually need to be concerned with trace gluten.

And keep in mind our gluten-free guideline: "If in doubt, go without." Do not eat a supposedly gluten-free food if there is no ingredient list or if you are not sure whether the ingredients are gluten-free. If you are unsure of the ingredients, call the food manufacturer for more information.

Finally, although the following list is reasonably comprehensive, it does not contain all the gluten-free foods being sold. And more gluten-free products are continually being developed and found on store shelves.

**Baking Mixes, etc**: Any baking mix you buy should be labeled "gluten-free." Most baking supplies, such as baking soda, sugar and cocoa, are considered gluten-free, but check ingredients to make certain. Davis, Rumford, Bob's Red Mill and Clabber Girl's baking powder are gluten free.
**All Purpose Flour**: Bob's Red Mill, King Arthur and other mills make gluten-free all-purpose flour.
**Corn Meal**:  Corn meal should be safe but check the label carefully.  Bob's Red Mill makes corn meal in gluten-free factory.
**Pancake Mix**: Bob's Red Mill, King Arthur, Bisquick and others make gluten free pancake mix.
**Pizza Dough**: Bob's Red Mill and King Arthur also make gluten free pizza dough.

**Bread Products**: The gluten in wheat, barley and rye consists of two proteins that combine during the baking process to form a substance that provides bread and other baked goods with elasticity and structure. Gluten also helps bread dough rise into a light, airy loaf.  Other grains do not have these characteristics, which is why it is difficult to find passable gluten-free bread. These days many supermarkets stock gluten-free bread, but you often can find a better selection online.
**Bread**: Udi's Whole Grain Bread (65 Calories per slice), Udi's White Sandwich Bread (70 Calories per slice) and Udi's Cinnamon Raisin Bread (70 Calories per slice), as well as many others are gluten free.
**Bread Crumbs**: Kinnikinnick Panko-Style Bread Crumbs are gluten free.

**Chow Mein Noodles**:  Goldberg's makes GF chow mein noodles.  They are sold in Walmart and many supermarkets.

**Hamburger Buns**: Kinnikinnick's Hamburger Buns (150 Calories), Rudi's Multi-Grain Hamburger Buns (190 Calories) and Udi's Classic and Whole-Grain Hamburger Buns (190 and 180 Calories per bun) are all gluten free.

**Hot Dog Buns**: Kinnikinnick's Hot Dog Buns (150 Calories), Rudi's Multi-Grain Hot Dog Buns (140 Calories) and Udi's Classic and Whole-Grain Hot Dog Buns (190 Calories) are all gluten free.

**Pita Bread**: Toufayan (110 Calories) sells gluten-free wraps.

**Polenta**: Bob's Red Mill Gluten Free Corn Grits/Polenta is gluten free.

: Some major brands now make several gluten-free cereals:
- General Mills Rice Chex (100 Calories per cup)
- General Mills Corn Chex (120 Calories per cup)
- General Mills Vanilla Chex (120 Calories per ¾ cup)
- General Mills Cinnamon Chex (120 Calories per ¾ cup)
- General Mills Chocolate Chex (130 Calories per ¾ cup)
- General Mills Apple Cinnamon Chex (130 Calories per ¾ cup)
- General Mills Honey Nut Chex (120 Calories per ¾ cup)
- Glutino Honey Nut (120 Calories per ¾ cup)
- Glutino Apple Cinnamon (120 Calories per ¾ cup).
- Kellogg's Rice Krispies - gluten-free (110 Calories per cup)
- Cream of Rice (150 Calories per packet)
- Bob's Red Mill Oat Meal
- GF Harvest Oat Meal (150 Calories per ½ cup)
- Waffles: Van's makes six varieties of gluten free waffles.

, **Fruit Drinks and Alcohol**: Unflavored coffee and black or green tea should be gluten-free, but flavored varieties may not be.  Most popular sodas in the United States are gluten-free.  Juice that is 100 percent fruit should be gluten-free, but fruit drinks made from fruit plus other ingredients may not be.  Conventional beer contains gluten; whereas, wine is gluten-free.

: In most cases, you will need to check ingredients or call the manufacturer to determine whether their product is gluten free.

**BBQ sauces:** Sweet Baby Ray's BBQ Sauce (35 Calories per tablespoon any variety), and KC Masterpiece BBQ Sauce (30 Calories per tablespoon any variety) are gluten free.

**Cajun Herb-Spice Mix**: Cajun's Choice Blackened and Creole Seasoning, Cajun Quick Shake Seasonings and McCormick's Cajun Seasoning are gluten free.

**Herb's & Spices**: . Regular salt and pepper should be gluten-free.  Fresh herbs and spices in a store's produce section are safe.  McCormick's single ingredient spices are gluten-free to 20 parts per million and their spice blends like Italian Seasoning and Salad Supreme Seasoning are gluten free.  Check other spice manufacturers for possible gluten cross-contamination.

**Marinades**: Bone Suckin' Original (also Poultry, Seafood & Steak) Seasoning & Rub and Kikkoman Gluten-Free Teriyaki Marinade & Sauce.

**Mustard & Ketchup**: French's yellow mustard and Heinz ketchup are gluten-free.

**Salsas:** The following salsas are gluten free to 20 ppm.  All varieties have 5 to 8 Calories per tablespoon.
- Amy's Salsa (mild & medium)
- Amy's Black Bean & Corn
- Farmer's Garden Salsa (medium & hot)
- Farmer's Peach
- Farmer's Pineapple
- Farmer's Roasted Garlic
- Newman's Own Black Bean & Corn
- Ortega Black Bean & Corn
- Ortega Garden Vegetable
- Ortega Original
- Ortega Thick & Chunky
- Ortega Salsa Verde

**Soy Sauce**: San-J and Kikkoman make gluten-free soy sauce.

**Tomato Sauce**: The following tomato sauces are both gluten free and low calorie:
- Classico Tomato & Basil Sauce (90 Calories per cup)
- Prego Light Smart Italian Sauce (90 Calories per cup)
- Hunt's Tomato Sauces (80 Calories per cup).

**Tomato Paste**: Hunt's is gluten free.

**Canned Tomatoes**:  Most canned tomatoes are safe including (but not limited to) Hunt's, Del Monte and Contadina.

**Vinegar:**  Distilled vinegar is derived from gluten grains but usually tests below the 20 ppm gluten threshold and is generally considered safe.  Quite a few people with celiac and gluten sensitivity, however, report that they react to both distilled vinegar and distilled alcohol.  To be safe, look for cider or balsamic vinegar rather than distilled vinegar.

**Worcestershire Sauce**: Lea & Perrins and French's Worcestershire Sauce are gluten free.  Read the ingredients to make sure nothing has changed.

**Cookies & Energy Bars**: There are quite a few good tasting gluten-free cookies on the market:
- Glutino's Chocolate Chip cookies, about 60 Calories each
- Glutino's Chocolate Vanilla Creme cookies, about 60 Calories each
- Glutino's Vanilla Creme cookies, about 65 Calories each
- Kinnikinnick's Ginger Snap cookies, about 40 Calories each
- Udi's Chocolate Chip cookies, about 95 Calories each
- Udi's Ginger cookies, about 90 Calories each
- Udi's Oatmeal Raisin cookies, about 90 Calories each
- Udi's Snicker Doodle cookies, about 90 Calories each

**Energy Bars:**  An energy bar is a convenient and sometimes healthy snack. But be careful to choose a brand that comes with protein, vitamins, and minerals, rather than high fructose, corn syrup or sugar. The following are five gluten-free energy bar manufacturers. (There are others.)
- Bumble Bar Organic Energy Bar (about 200 Calories per bar)
- Macrobars Organic Peanut Protein (about 260 Calories)
- NuGo 10 Raw Natural Energy Bar (200 Calories)
- Pure Organic Raw Fruit & Nut Bar (about 200 Calories)
- Raw Revolution Organic Food Bar (about 230 Calories).

**Frozen Entrees**: Most larger supermarkets have a reasonably good selection of frozen entrees.  At this writing, Amy's and Artisan Bistro sell more gluten-free frozen entrees than any other manufacturer.  Smart Ones makes two gluten-free entrees.  Glutino offers two gluten-free frozen entrees, although each contain 400 Calories, and are not included in the following list.
- Amy's Black Bean & Cheese Enchilada (240 Calories)
- Amy's Mushroom Risotto Bowl (240 Calories)
- Amy's Quinoa & Black Beans w Butternut Squash & Chard (240 Calories)
- Amy's Sweet & Sour Asian Noodle Bowl (250 Calories)
- Amy's Vegetable Parmesan Bowl (260 Calories)
- Amy's Brown Rice & Veggies Bowl – Light in Sodium (260 Calories)
- Amy's Teriyaki Bowl (290 Calories)
- Amy's Brown Rice, Black-eyed Peas & Veggies Bowl (290 Calories)
- Amy's Asian Noodle Stir Fry (300 Calories)
- Amy's Vegetable Lasagna (300 Calories)
- Amy's Thai Stir-Fry (310 Calories)
- Amy's Tofu Scramble (320 Calories)

- Artisan Bistro Chicken Parmesan Bake (200 Calories)

- Artisan Bistro Wild Alaskan Salmon (200 Calories)
- Artisan Bistro Turkey Cheddar Bake (240 Calories)
- Artisan Bistro Thai Style Yellow Curry with Chicken (240 Calories)
- Artisan Bistro Wild Alaskan Salmon Bake (240 Calories)
- Artisan Bistro Cheddar Beef Bake (250 Calories)
- Artisan Bistro Sesame Ginger with Salmon (270 Calories)
- Artisan Bistro Spiced Chicken Morocco (270 Calories)
- Artisan Bistro Coconut Lemongrass with Chicken (270 Calories)
- Artisan Bistro Thai Style Red Curry with Beef (280 Calories)
- Artisan Bistro Albacore Tuna Bake (280 Calories)
- Artisan Bistro Chicken Citron (280 Calories)
- Artisan Bistro Wild Alaskan Salmon with Pesto (310 Calories)
- Artisan Bistro Savory Turkey (330 Calories)
- Artisan Bistro Southwest Style Beef (330 Calories)
- Artisan Bistro Ginger Chicken (350 Calories)
- Artisan Bistro Beef with Mushroom Sauce (350 Calories)
- Artisan Bistro Wild Alaskan Salmon Cake (370 Calories)

- Smart Ones Lemon Herb Chicken Piccata (250 Calories)
- Smart Ones Santa Fe Style Rice & Beans (290 Calories)

**Fruits and Vegetables**:  Fresh fruits, berries, greens and vegetables are naturally gluten free and generally safe. Most canned fruits and vegetables are gluten-free, but some are not.  Single-ingredient frozen fruits and vegetables are generally gluten free, but frozen fruits and vegetables with multiple ingredients frequently contain gluten.  Generally, more ingredients in a food increase the chance for trace gluten.  Read labels carefully or contact the manufacturer to determine if a particular product is processed in a factory or on manufacturing lines shared with gluten-containing products.

**Legumes and Rice**:  Legumes (lentils, beans, etc) are naturally gluten free, but there is always the risk of cross-contamination during processing and handling.  And be wary of canned lentils, beans, etc that have added ingredients.  "If in doubt, go without."

Brown Rice, white rice, long-grained rice, sticky rice and wild rice are all naturally gluten-free.

**Meat, Poultry & Fish**: Fresh meat, poultry and fish generally are safe on a gluten-free diet if they are not gluten cross-contaminated at a supermarket or butcher shop.  (Realize that the display cases in many stores contain fans that circulate air that could cross-contaminate unprotected meat, poultry and fish. When in doubt choose meat, poultry and fish covered in plastic wrap.)

On the other hand, packaged processed meats, such as hams, bacon, sausages and luncheon meats, could contain gluten.  Look for packaged processed meat products labeled gluten-free.  Beware of meats and poultry with added ingredients that make them  ready-to-cook meals.  Most are not safe on a gluten-free diet because the store might have used unsafe ingredients when repackaging the food.  Avoid these products.

There are plenty of gluten-free **deli meats**. All of Boar's Head's products are gluten-free and Hormel and Hillshire Farms both make packaged gluten-free meats. But be wary of cross-contamination by shared slicing machines at the deli counter. To make sure deli meat or cheese are gluten free, choose pre-packaged products.

There are lots of **hams** that are considered gluten-free to 20 ppm, although most are not labeled gluten-free. Again check with the manufacturer.

GF **bacon** is widely available. A partial list includes:  Applegate Farms, Boar's Head, Jones Dairy Farm, and Wellshire Farms.  The following is a partial list of low-calorie gluten-free bacon: Jones Turkey Bacon (35 Calories per slice) and Wellshire Farms Turkey Bacon (40 Calories per slice).

Many **hot dogs** are gluten-free, and a few are labeled gluten-free.  A partial list follows: Jennie-O Turkey Franks (95 Calories each), Applegate Chicken Hot Dog (60 Calories each) and Turkey Hot Dog (50 Calories each).

The following is a partial listing of GF **burger patties**: Jennie-O Turkey Burgers (200 Calories each), Applegate Turkey Burgers (140 Calories each) and Beef Burgers (195 Calories each).

GF **veggie burgers** are produced by Amy's, Dr Praeger's and others: Amy's Bistro Veggie Burger (110 Calories) and Sonoma Veggie Burger (140 Calories) and Dr. Praeger's California Veggie Burger (110 Calories).

Many **sausages** contain bread crumbs as a filler, so check labels carefully before buying. In addition, even if the sausage does not include a gluten ingredient, it may have been manufactured on equipment that also processes gluten-containing sausage. The following is a partial list of GF sausage manufacturers: Al Fresco, Applegate Farms, Jones Dairy Farm, Smithfield and Wellshire Farms. (We just tested an Al Fresco chicken sausage, and found it to be tasty, low calorie and gluten-free.  Al Fresco sausages are sold in many supermarkets.)

Canned **tuna and salmon** produced by Chicken of the Sea and by Bubble Bee are gluten free.

**Milk and Dairy Products**: Most milk and many dairy-based products are gluten-free.  Plain, unflavored milk, butter, plain yogurt, fresh eggs and many cheeses are gluten-free. Some ice creams are gluten-free.  And many flavored yogurts are gluten-free. Check the ingredients to be sure.

**Milk Substitutes:**  Soy, rice and almond milk are most often gluten-free, but some are not.  Check the labels.  (Soy, rice and almond milk may be substituted for cow's skim milk provided the calorie count is close.)
**Yogurt**:  All varieties of Chobani and Yoplait yogurt, including flavored varieties, are gluten free.  Yoplait Light in the 6 oz container has 90 Calories.
**Cheeses**: Most cheeses are naturally gluten-free.  One slice (1 oz) of light cheese has about 70 Calories. Beware of cheese that has been sliced and repackaged at a supermarket.  It might be cross contaminated.  Usually, it is safer to buy cheese that has been packaged at the manufacturer's plant.
**Cottage Cheese**: Breakstone, Cabot, Humboldt and others make fat free, gluten-free cottage cheese.
**Ice Cream**: Although many ice cream products are gluten free, some are not.  Also consider GF frozen fruit pops. All of Skinny Cow's ice cream bars are gluten free: Chocolate Truffle Bar (100 Calories), Caramel Truffle Bar (100 Calories) and Fudge Bars (110 Calories).

**Oils, Nuts & Popcorn**:  Most oils (olive, canola, etc), nuts, and popcorn varieties are gluten free.  Nuts are naturally gluten free.  But beware of nuts and popcorn with added flavorings that might contain gluten.  Some popcorn brands that are considered gluten free are Jolly Time, Newman's Own and Orville Redenbacher's.
**Peanut Butter**: Arrowhead Mills and Smart Balance peanut butter are gluten free (about 95 Calories per tablespoon.)
**Mayonnaise**:  Hellmann's and Best Foods regular and light mayonnaise are gluten free. (light is 35 Calories per serving)
**Non-Stick Cooking Spray**: Original Pam, Mazola and Wegman's store brand cooking sprays are gluten free.

**Pasta**: Fortunately, there are a number of gluten-free pastas available, in different shapes and sizes.  Choose gluten-free pasta made from rice or corn rather than wheat. Surprisingly, many of these gluten-free varieties are quite good, making it possible to serve gluten-free pasta whose taste is very close to wheat-based pasta.  The following manufacturers make gluten-free pasta: Ancient Harvest, Andean Dream, Bionaturae, Jovial, DeBoles, DeLallo, Le Veneziane, Lundberg, Riso Bello, Rizopia, Ronzoni, Rustichella D'Abruzzo, Sam Mills and Tinkyada.

**Salad Dressings**: When buying vinaigrette-type salad dressings look for cider or balsamic vinegar, not distilled vinegar on the food label. (Distilled vinegar is made from gluten grains.)  The following salad dressings are gluten free:
- Annie's Lite Raspberry Vinaigrette (20 Calories per tablespoon)

- Annie's Lite Italian Dressing (23 Calories per tablespoon)
- Annie's Lite Honey Mustard Vinaigrette (20 Calories per tablespoon)
- Annie's Lite Herb Balsamic Vinaigrette (25 Calories per tablespoon)
- Annie's Lite Gingerly Vinaigrette (20 Calories per tablespoon).
- Gazebo Room Lite Greek Salad Dressing (20 Calories per tablespoon)
- Ken's Lite Options Italian w/ Romano & Red Pepper (23 Calorie per tablespoon)
- Newman's Own Lite Balsamic Vinaigrette (13 Calorie per tablespoon)
- Newman's Own Lite Roasted Garlic Balsamic (25 Calories per tablespoon)
- Newman's Own Lite Red Wine Vinaigrette & Olive Oil (25 Calories per tablespoon)
- Newman's Own Lite Low-Fat Sesame Ginger (18 Calories per tablespoon)
- San-J's Tamari Sesame Salad Dressing (20 Calories per tablespoon)
- San-J's Tamari Ginger Salad Dressing (13 Calories per tablespoon)
- Sophia's Oil-Free Cilantro & Lime (5 Calories per tablespoon)

**Soups**  **(See Appendix C for a list of GF soup.)**
Amy's Kitchen: A great many of Amy's 29 soups are considered gluten-free to 20 ppm.
Bookbinders Specialties: This gourmet soup company has 11 gluten-free soups. All are tested to below 20 ppm, and are available by mail order or in U.S. supermarkets in the northeast.
Frontier Soup:  Frontier makes 28 varieties of gluten-free soup mixes.  All are certified to below 5ppm of gluten.  Frontier Soup mixes are available online and at upscale supermarket chains.
Imagine Foods:  Imagine Foods claims all varieties of its soups are gluten-free to 20 ppm except for Organic Creamy Chicken and Imagine Bistro Bisques.  Imagine soups are usually found in the "natural foods" section of supermarkets.
Pacific Foods:  Almost all Pacific's soups are gluten free. Most often Pacific soups are found in the natural or health food section of a supermarket, although in some stores they are next to conventional soups.
Progresso: Choose from Progresso's many gluten-fee varieties tested to 20 ppm.

**Stock, Broth & Bouillon**:  Stock is made by simmering vegetables, bones, meat scraps, etc, and is the best base for soups, stews, and sauces. Unfortunately stock is rarely found on supermarket shelves.  Broth is stock with added salt and can be used in the same way as homemade stock -- although broth is not as rich and complex as stock.  Bouillon is dehydrated stock formed into cubes or granules.  It is convenient but is typically processed with large amounts of sodium and other additives.  Thus the liquid it produces is almost flavorless.

Kitchen Basics makes gluten free Chicken, Beef, Vegetable, Turkey, Seafood, Veal, Unsalted Chicken and Unsalted Beef stock.  Pacific Foods sells gluten free vegetable broth, mushroom broth, beef broth and chicken and vegetable stock.  College Inn's garden-vegetable broth, organic-beef broth, tender-beef bold stock and white wine & herb broth are all considered gluten-free to 20ppm.  Hormel's vegetable, beef and chicken bouillon cubes are gluten free.

**Miscellaneous**
We put food products in this category that did not seem to fit anywhere else. Pancake Syrup: Hungry Jack Lite Syrup (25 Calories per tablespoon ), Log Cabin Lite Syrup (25 Calories per tablespoon) and Vermont Maid Lite Syrup (30 Calories per tablespoon) are gluten free.

# Appendix C
# Gluten-Free Soup

| Soup Description | Calories* |
|---|---|
| Amy's Vegetable Barley Soup | 70 |
| Progresso Chicken Rice with Vegetables Soup | 80 |
| Amy's Alphabet Soup | 80 |
| Pacific Chicken Noodle Soup | 90 |
| Progresso Vegetable Classics Garden Vegetable Soup | 90 |
| Amy's Split Pea Soup | 100 |
| Pacific Butternut Squash Bisque | 110 |
| Amy's Cream of Tomato Soup | 110 |
| Progresso Traditional Manhattan Clam Chowder | 110 |
| Pacific Roasted Red Pepper & Tomato Soup | 110 |
| Amy's Mushroom Bisque with Porcini | 120 |
| Amy's Pasta & 3 Bean Soup | 130 |
| Pacific Chicken Spinach Penne Soup | 140 |
| Amy's Hearty Minestrone with Vegetables Soup | 150 |
| Amy's Summer Corn & Vegetable Soup | 150 |
| Progresso Vegetable Classics Lentil Soup | 160 |
| Amy's Tuscan Bean & Rice Soup | 160 |
| Progresso Hearty New England Clam Chowder | 180 |
| Progresso Potato Broccoli & Cheese Chowder | 200 |

See page 47 for additional gluten-free soup manufacturers.

*** Important:** Calories per serving. When the Daily Meal Plan menu specifies soup, have only one serving (8 ounces) unless stated otherwise. (Note cans of soup usually contain about two servings.)

# Appendix D
# Exercise Smart

Our bodies are just not built to be immobile and passive. The sad fact, however, is that after years of education and information programs by government agencies, medical associations   and  insurance companies, relatively few  Americans  engage in  regular
planned exercise – despite the reality that we need to be active to keep our systems working efficiently and rid ourselves of emotional tension. Moreover, exercise burns calories, speeds up your metabolism and is an invaluable part of any weight control program.  There are two ways to become more physically active: 1) Increase the physical activity in your daily life; and 2) Start on a regular exercise program.  Better still would be a combination of both. Simply stated there are three basic types of exercise: aerobic, stretching and strengthening.

**Aerobic Exercises** (also called "cardio") condition your cardiovascular system. Aerobic exercises, such as jogging, swimming, cycling, brisk walking, skipping rope, and many others, are typically deep breathing and continuous, with rhythmic and repetitive contractions of your large muscle groups. The trait most aerobic exercises have in common is that they make you work hard and require you process a great deal of oxygen.

Some typical aerobic exercises are:  Most strenuous include bicycling, cross-country skiing, dancing (aerobic), hiking in rugged terrain, ice hockey, jogging, jogging in place, rowing, skipping rope, stair climbing, and stationary cycling.  Somewhat less strenuous are basketball, field hockey, calisthenics, handball, racquetball, skiing (downhill), soccer, squash, tennis (singles), volleyball, and walking (briskly). Least strenuous aerobic exercises consist of badminton, baseball, bowling, croquet, dancing, gardening, golf (carrying or pulling clubs), horseback riding, housework, ping-pong, shuffleboard, softball, tennis (doubles) and walking (moderate to leisurely).

**Stretching-type Exercises** such as yoga, tai chi, Pilates and to a lesser extent calisthenics can improve your flexibility – and some of the exercises can make you somewhat stronger.

As you age you inevitably start to loose flexibility. Your gait becomes stiffer; you can't stand quite as upright as you used to; it becomes tougher to bend over; and you have difficulty turning your neck. Regardless of your age, however, stretching can make you more flexible, less injury prone, and can reduce the pain and discomfort associated with tight muscles and shortened tendons. Realize, however, that stretching exercises do not condition your heart and lungs. Stretching exercises are fine as long as they are performed in addition to rather than in place of an aerobic exercise.

Most experts do recommend stretching before and after an aerobic or strength routine. However, never stretch cold muscles and always do some form of warm up prior to stretching.  Stretch slowly and hold gently. You should stretch to the point of feeling a mild pull, but you should never feel pain.  And when you stretch – do not bounce.

**Muscle Building and Strengthening** Exercises, e.g., weight lifting, use of the machines found in fitness centers and isometrics.

Once more, as you age you loose muscle mass, your bone density decreases and you lose strength. Exercises like weight lifting strengthen your muscles, bones and joints. Strengthening exercises also reduce your risk of developing osteoporosis, a severe bone-loss disease, which can lead to easily fractured bones and all the complications that often follow. Strong muscles not only allow you to lift a sleepy four-year old out of a car without difficulty and lug groceries up to a second floor apartment, but as with increased flexibility, strong muscles also make you less injury prone. Moreover, because **muscle uses many more calories than fat, when you replace fat with muscle, your metabolism actually speeds up.**

For everything you need to know about exercise see *Exercises Smart - U.S. Edition*, an eBook by Earl Simmons also published by NoPaperPress.

# NoPaperPress Paperbacks and eBooks

100-Day Super Diet-1200 Calorie*
100-Day Super Diet-1500 Calorie*
100-Day No-Cooking Diet-1200 Cal*
100-Day No-Cooking Diet-1500 Cal*
90-Day Smart Diet-1200 Calorie*
90-Day Smart Diet-1500 Calorie*
90-Day No-Cooking Diet - 1200 Cal*
90-Day No-Cooking Diet - 1500 Cal*
90-Day Perfect Diet - 1200 Calorie*
90-Day Perfect Diet - 1500 Calorie*
60-Day Perfect Diet-1200 Calorie*
60-Day Perfect Diet-1500 Calorie*
50-Day Flex Diet-1200 Calorie*
50-Day Flex Diet-1500 Calorie*
30-Day Quick Diet - for Women*
30-Day Quick Diet - for Men*
30-Day No-Cooking Diet*
30-Day Diet for Women - Metric*
30-Day Diet for Men - Metric*
25 Day Easy Diet-1200 Calorie*
25 Day Easy Diet-1500 Calorie*
25-Day No-Cooking Diet
10-Day Express Diet
10-Day No-Cooking Diet*
7-Day Diet for Women*
7-Day Diet for Men*
7-Day No-Cooking Diets*
90-Day Gluten-Free Diet-1200 Cal*
90-Day Gluten-Free Diet-1500 Cal*
30-Day Gluten-Free Quick Diet*
30-Day Gluten-Free No-Cooking Diet*
7-Day Diet for Women - Metric*
7-Day Diet for Men - Metric
7-Day Gluten-Free Express Diet*
7-Day Gluten-Free No-Cooking Diet*
90-Day Vegetarian Diet-1200 Calorie*
90-Day Vegetarian Diet-1500 Calorie*
30-Day Vegetarian Diet*
7-Day Vegetarian Diet*
Weight Loss for Women*
Weight Loss for Women - Metric
Weight Loss for Women - UK
Weight Loss for Men*
Maximum Weight Loss - 1200 Cal*
Maximum Weight Loss - 1500 Cal*

Weight Loss for Men - Metric*
Maximum Weight Loss- 1200 Calorie*
Maximum Weight Loss- 1500 Calorie*
Weight Control - U.S. Edition
Weight Control - Metric. Edition
Professional Weight Control Women - U.S.
Professional Weight Control Women - Metric
Professional Weight Control Men - U.S.
Professional Weight Control Men - Metric
Weight Maintenance - U.S. Edition*
Weight Maintenance - Metric. Edition*
Weight Maintenance - UK Edition
Weight Loss for Senior Men*
Weight Loss for Senior Women*
Eat Smart - U.S. Edition*
Eat Smart - Metric Edition
30-Day Mediterranean Diet
Exercise Smart - U.S. Edition*
Exercise Smart - Metric Edition
Exercise Smart - UK Edition*
Total Fitness - U.S. Edition
Total Fitness - Metric Edition
Total Fitness - UK Edition
Total Fitness for Women-U.S. Edition*
Total Fitness for Women - Metric
Total Fitness for Women - UK Edition
Total Fitness for Men - U.S. Edition*
Total Fitness for Men- Metric Edition*
Total Fitness for Men - UK Edition
Senior Fitness - U.S. Edition*
Senior Fitness - Metric Edition*
Senior Fitness - UK Edition*
Computer Diet - U.S. Edition*
Computer Diet - Metric Edition*
Reliable Weight Loss - U.S. Edition
101 Weight Loss Tips*
101 Healthy Eating Tips*
101 Lifelong Fitness Tips*
101 Weight Maintenance Tips
101 Weight Loss Recipes
101 Gluten-Free Weight Loss Recipes
101 Vegetarian Weight Loss Recipes*
30-Day Mediterranean Diet*
90-Day Mediterranean Diet - 1200 Cal*
90-Day Mediterranean Diet - 1500 Cal*

* These titles are available as both ebooks and paperbacks. Our ebooks are sold by Amazon, Apple, Google, Barnes & Noble and Kobo. But our paperbacks are only sold by Amazon.

# Disclaimer

This book offers general meal planning, nutrition and weight control information.  It is not a medical manual and the authors do not claim to be medically qualified.  Everyone should have a medical checkup before beginning this gluten-free weight loss program.  Moreover, the physician conducting the medical exam should be made aware of and should approve this diet.  Because commercial food ingredients and formulations can change at any time, adults with celiac disease or gluten sensitivity should be particularly careful and double check the ingredients in the foods listed in this book to be sure they are gluten free.  We recommend that you do not solely rely on the information presented here and that you always read labels, warnings, and directions before using or consuming a product.  For additional information about a product, please contact the manufacturer.  The content on this site is for reference purposes and is not intended to substitute for advice given by a physician, pharmacist, or other licensed health-care professional.  You should not use this information as self-diagnosis or for treating a health problem or disease.  Contact your health-care provider immediately if you suspect that you have a medical problem.  Additionally, while the authors and publisher have made every effort to ensure the accuracy of the information in this book, they make no representations or warranties regarding its accuracy or completeness.  Further, neither the authors nor publisher assume liability for any medical problems that might result from applying the methods in this book, or for any loss of profit, or any other commercial damages, including but not limited to special, incidental, consequential or other damages, and any such liability is hereby expressly disclaimed.

www.ingramcontent.com/pod-product-compliance
Lightning Source LLC
Chambersburg PA
CBHW051420250726
48655CB00003B/1142